I0414218

Ten Simple Steps to Permanent Weight Loss

Patricia Smith

Copyright © 2016

Table of Contents

Introduction

'Hey, you look slimmer than before! Have you lost weight?!' – is probably the best compliment that anyone can receive in today's world. If you agree, then you would understand that losing weight to remain fit and healthy is one of the most important concerns for everyone. It is not that we are all fat or overweight, it is just that somewhere along the way of following and believing in our dreams, we lose sight of what is most important to us – our health.

It is an oft-repeated line that makes complete sense now – Health is Wealth. No amount of riches in the world can replace out true gems – our health. What you need to remember is that just like how every book has its own owner every individual is the author of his own health.

Everybody needs some advice at some point in time in their lives. Let this be a constant motivation for all the times that you need some motivation to get fit. Peruse this book and you will be surprised that all it takes is a little effort and commitment from your side to ensure a successful and fit you. What you need is some determination and everyday inspiration to keep you going. The thing about gaining weight is that usually one does not even realize that he or she has put on weight until it begins to reflect in some way or the other things that we do or in some comments.

It is true that unlike men, women are very obsessed with their weights and many cannot stop checking the weighing machine on a daily basis after registering for a weight loss program.

Chapter 1: How To Lose Weight?

Weight loss may seem like a very difficult task at the outset. Hence, we advise you to follow the series of steps and think about how these tips will enhance the weight loss program. Do not jump into any program without debating the pros and cons.

Tip 1: Be proactive and Think positive

Given that there is a world of difference between being slim and acting like you are fit, the focus of these diets should extend to a sort of worry In all aspects of life. There are two ways of looking at food – how heavy it may make you feel or how light it could possibly be. People on the heavier side of the weighing scales tend to imagine how food is going to taste

Every time that you are tempted to do something along the lines of binge eating, take a hard look at your priorities and decide what works best for you. It is also a good idea to surround yourself with slim people who eat less and are fitness conscious individuals.

Tip 2: Be fair, be practical

Motivation is something that one needs to develop on a daily basis. You may keep doing everything right and you can still get that one day when you feel like it is not your cup of tea. You may come so close to quitting that you actually do your fitness regime because it is beyond you reach. It is in these moments that you want to give up and it is a tough time. One weak moment is enough to induce guilt and make you do something you regret.

Tip 3: Weight loss is not a cure-all solution

Many people believe that when they become slimmer and fitter, they will stop having everyday problems. This is definitely not true. It's true that there are perks to looking and feeling good but there are times when every individual goes through unexpected moments and they may affect you during your moments of self-doubt, or at those miserable moments when you feel undervalued. If you are someone who fixed high hopes on being thin and discovered it does not solve your problems and began eating again, then it is best to stay away from junk during these moments. Losing weight is a truly big achievement but maintaining your weight can also be doubly hard, more so because you have to resist eating all those things that you were hitherto banned from eating.

Tip 4: Only eat when you're hungry

There is no better feeling in the world than when you are eating good food when you are really hungry. Ensure that you stay away from extreme carbohydrates because eating sugary foods can cause a subsequent crash in energy, leaving you wanting more sweetness. If you want to eat something quite filling, then opt for slow energy release food items, which are usually the likes of protein. It is a good habit to eat protein with every meal alongside 'good carbs' such as whole grains, vegetables, fruits, and beans because this will help in avoiding the 'crash and burn' of sugar overdosing.

The lifestyle today is a little skewed and people are gaining weight at a faster pace than ever before. Here are a few trends that we analyze:

- Presence of chemicals in food

It is true that almost all our vegetables and fruits are grown in pesticide-laden fields. There are very few organic farmers out there who make a decent living. These pesticides or insecticides are actually chemicals that have the power to cause weight gain. You must make it a habit to wash the produce in salted water or vinegar. It is best to soak it in a vessel and allow the toxins to come off the skin.

- Harmful Smell

A lot of industrial solvents have a horrible stench attached which may not seem so bad at that time. However, it is not a good idea to remain exposed to the smells of nail polish remover, glues, paints or varnishes.

- Stress

Although people associate stress with weight loss, there are numerous cases when being overworked and tired may cause weight gain. This is because stress makes you want to look for comfort outside of your body and you usually find it in the foods that you eat. In women, stress also decreases the output of progesterone. One needs to eat well and sleep well in order to be fit.

Chapter 2: How To Go About Achieving Permanent Weight Loss?

- Set Goals

Setting goals is the most important step when it comes to losing weight. You need to know what you are getting into and be reminded of it constantly. After planning a goal, you will now decide how to go about it? Should you cut all the sugar from your diet? Should you try portion control? Eliminate everything and go on a detox diet? Depending on your body weight and eating habits, we will need to figure out a diet plan that is exclusive to you. Copying the diets of your friends will not help you in this regard in any way.

You could also attempt to use smaller sized plates. You may automatically end up eating less because your portions are less – it may look fuller than it already is.

- Track things

To begin the process, you can create a food diary wherein you write out your day's intake of food. Identify the likely culprits that are causing havoc to your health. These might usually be soft drinks, juices, chocolate, muffins and confectionery. It may seem like a tedious job but you will need to eliminate these from your foodstuffs to lose the kilos. Healthy eating and healthy living can only be possible if you are extremely motivated for the same thing. You have got to be self-aware and accountable. Keep a food diary and exercise log to record your daily intake. This will help you where you may be mistakenly going wrong with the calories count.

- Do not Cut All Food

Eating healthy diets requires you to eat in moderation – nothing is forbidden but you still cannot go overboard and munch on those cookies simply because you are bored and have nothing to do. All form of mindless eating needs to be stopped the minute you decide to take matters of the expanding waistline in your own hands. Also, ensure that you taste all the food that is present on the dining table but restrict the portion of the food that may be fattening.

- Stay Dedicated

It is crucial for you to be vigilant about what you eat and when. There may be many instances when you cannot help but reach out to that crispy potato wedges. If your mind makes you feel guilty about eating it, then you are on the right track. Stop eating the unhealthy food and quit it right then. Exercise makes weight loss a lot easier so whether you like it or not, you will have to start becoming a more active person.

- Get A Group

Support from your friends and families will make your journey into weight loss a lot less challenging because you will have someone to stand up to you and tell you when you falter. Be it your close-knit circle of friends or colleagues, if your co-workers are on the same page as you, then they will also be conscious of their eating habits when around you.

Chapter 3: Busting Metabolism Myths

It is true that one's metabolism slows with age but there are things that you can do to keep it going up and about. There are tricks to bring your metabolism up to task.

* Eat Enough

This may sound tricky coming at a point when we're all worried about the calories we consume but it is essential to eat enough food – more than the amount required for basic biological function. This amounts to about 1200 calories for most women. What happens if you eat lesser than this?

Chances are that the body begins to break down the calorie-burning muscle tissue for energy or precious other such processes. It is okay to snack between meal times because the period between breakfast and lunch or lunch and dinner can be extremely long and it may make you weak and hungry if you do not eat on time.

* Do not skip breakfast

Regardless of the time that you wake up (it is an added advantage if you do end up waking early, breakfast is the most important meal of the day and you should not skip it at any cost. There is a reason we have that popular saying that goes thus – 'Breakfast like a king, lunch like a common man, and dine like a pauper'. Studies indicate that women who skip breakfast are 4.5 times more likely to be obese. You do not have to fuss over what to eat, just make sure that you grab a yoghurt or oatmeal made with low-fat or fat-free meal if you do not have time for a full-fledged breakfast. Nuts are rich in essential minerals and vitamins so you can almost always top it up with whatever you need.

Chapter 4: What Happens to Your Body When You Consume Carbohydrates?

Carbohydrate-rich foods are those processed and packaged foodstuffs that we are exposed to on a daily basis. These can include dry cereal, crackers, rice cakes, etc which convert the carbohydrates to simple sugars and send it directly into the blood stream. There is always some extra insulin produced by the pancreas, which helps your body absorb the sugar that is contained in all these food items at the soonest opportunity possible. Because of the sugar rush and the immediate conversion of sugar into energy, you may soon end up with low blood sugar and then hunger pangs continue. When this happens, then you may be inclined to reach for the same kind of sugary foods with no nutritional value again to satisfy your need for instant energy, and thus, the vicious cycle continues. Make sure that you read the labels of all the products that you consume – more often than not, even the health supplements or foods are rich in sugar, but they claim to be healthy on account of the presence of other substances.

I am not suggesting that you cut off the carbohydrates entirely! That is definitely not the focus of this section. Instead, we shall understand what you must do and how. What you need to understand is that the snacks containing a rich combination of carbohydrates, healthy fats, and protein take a longer time to digest. This also includes frozen food items that are laden with sodium, a natural preservative. The thing with sodium is that it makes your body retain water, which bloats you up. So, in conclusion, so you won't look and feel your best regardless of how much weight you want to lose.

Chapter 5: Understanding Healthy Eating Habits

Weight loss paranoia reigns supreme in the globalized world that even the simplest food items get ignored. Here's a look at some of the less stressed upon food and drink that we all are aware of. Let us take a moment to understand how or why they are important and what the effects of these are in our body.

- Hot Beverages Are Welcome

According to a study conducted by the Japanese, a cup of brewed tea can actually help increase your metabolism by up to 12 percent. If you are a coffee addict like me, then feel free to have the warm stimulant without many doubts because caffeine can jolt your metabolism up to 8%, making you burn calories at a faster rate. Just remember to avoid too much sugar in your beverages.

Green tea is another beverage that you can add to the list – it is healthy and also rich in antioxidants that claim to promote weight loss extensively. The antioxidants present in green tea are called catechins that work on the fat cells and help you lose some pounds.

- Use Coconut Oil While Cooking

We are all used to the idea of using vegetable or sunflower oil for cooking out food. Little do we realize that the healthier oil would be olive or coconut oil. Coconut oil is rich in fat such as medium chain triglycerides that are metabolized differently as compared to fats.

- Fibre is Fab

Consuming a solid proportion of fibre is good for your body as it can burn as much as thirty percent fat in your body. Vegetables are a good source of fibre. This not only boosts your metabolism but it works wonders on your digestion as well. Eating fibre as a part of your meal will ensure that you gain the least amount of weight over time.

- Drink Plenty Of Water

If you drink up to 48 ounces of water, then the German researches estimate that it will increase your metabolism by up to 50 calories daily. Apparently this could be due to the fact that the temperature of the water will need to be increased to match the body temperature.

- Organic Is Awesome

Pesticides that we unknowingly consume the food that we eat may contain toxic substances that trigger weight gain. It is always better to choose organic items when buying fruits and vegetables to avoid falling into this trap.

- Protein is powerful

It is a must to include protein in your everyday diet instead of carbs or fats. You can vary your proteins and alternate between low-fat yoghurt, lean meat, nuts, fish, etc.

- Iron Is Essential

Besides proteins, it is a good idea to consume iron-rich food such as shellfish, beans, egg-plant, apple etc. Not only does this help your hemoglobin levels, but the overall energy of your body is affected too. Lack of iron often causes anaemia in women. Spinach and fortified cereals are also rich in iron and you can think of innovative ways to which you can add these to your diets to supplement your nutrition.

Iron is especially important for women because women lose iron each month during menstruation. Low iron presence in the body can sap your energy and leave you with a sagging metabolism.

- Vitamin D content

Vitamin D is crucial for preserving metabolism-revving muscle tissue. Research reveals that only about 4% of Americans over age 50 get enough vitamin D through their diet. Besides the early morning sun, you can get the right amount of Vitamin D by choosing food items such as salmon, tuna, shrimp, tofu, fortified milk and cereal, or eggs.

- Limit Alcohol Content

Alcohol causes you to burn fat at a slower rate and it can reduce your body's fat-burning ability by up to 73%. Instead of opting for a series of cocktails or beers, just stick to fruit juices or water and allow your body to remain toxin free. If you are an avid beer lover, then you will have to be extra careful because a lot of people complain of beer bellies once they begin drinking. This may be due to the fact that consuming alcohol tends to make you hungry and due to which you may end up eating a lot more than you intended to.

Alcohol does not support weight loss and if you are high then your judgement about what food to eat and which to stay away from may be impaired. Hence, one drink party is enough to set you back with a lot more calories on. When there is alcohol present in the body, the sole focus of the liver is on the alcohol – it wants to eliminate the toxin at the soonest because of its detox mode, thus, the fat-burning ability suffers.

- Milk is Mandatory

Low levels of calcium in your blood and bones may not help your cause when you are attempting to lose weight. A lack of calcium can cause slow metabolism and reduce fat absorption from other foods. As kids, we all go through the phase of being forced to drink milk. As we grow older, our lifestyle choices and supplements barely include drinking milk but this trend needs to change. Calcium is particularly important to women during the menopausal age. If you hate drinking milk in itself, try hot chocolate or flavored milk so as to get the required levels of calcium in your body.

- What's the secret of those high-fibre snack bars?

We have talked aplenty about the importance of fibre in our diets but this does not mean that we end up consuming processed fibre. No, indeed not. What you must focus on is including some natural fibre - any fruit or vegetable. This can be a light meal in itself during the course of your day. Bananas are a great source of potassium and fibre and it will elevate your blood sugar levels immediately.

- Not All Low-Fat Foods Are Healthy

What happens when fat is removed from the food is that it becomes less tasty as the flavor of the food is gone so the producers end up adding more sugar to the food which is disastrous for those trying to lose weight. People also assume that the food is good for them and eat more than is healthy for people.

Chapter 6: What Should You Eat?

One must concentrate on equal and healthy proportions of the meal so as to enable a balanced diet. Here's a look at some of the foodstuffs that actually complement your diet and help you on the way to losing those kilos.

- Whole Eggs

Eggs are normally high in protein and this is their USP. They can be made in a variety of ways and are good for the body whether it is boiled, poached or scrambled. They also have the ability to make one feel full after consumption.

- Leafy Greens

Whether it is spinach, kale or collards, green leaves are rich in fibre and make for interesting meals. They are low in both fat and carbohydrate content and it increases the volume of the meals without increasing the calories. They are nutritious because they contain a good amount of vitamins, minerals and antioxidants. This includes calcium, which has been shown to aid fat burning.

- Fish

Oily fish like salmon are incredibly healthy when you are health conscious. Fish is rich in proteins and it is loaded with omega 3 acids that are not found in any other mean. What's more, it is also very satisfying and keeps you full for many hours with relatively few calories. Seafood in general is rich in iodine content. Iodine is a must for the proper functioning of the thyroid gland, which is also important to keep the metabolism running optimally high. The omega 3 fatty acids reduce inflammation, which is known to play a major role in obesity and metabolic disease. You can try different types of fish such as mackerel, trout, sardines and herring for variety in this department. Tuna is another great food that is high in protein and low on calories. It is a lean fish and is very popular among bodybuilders and fitness models. Just remember to choose tuna canned in water, but not oil.

- Cruciferous Veggies

High in fibre and yet filling in nature. Cruciferous vegetables like cauliflower, cabbage, broccoli and brussels sprouts contain decent amounts of protein compared to most vegetables.

- Meat

Meat is a weight loss friendly food, because of its high protein value. Eating a high protein diet can make you burn up to 80 to 100 more calories per day. What's more, recent studies have shown that increasing your protein intake to 25-30% of calories can also cut cravings by 60%.

- Potato Power

Potatoes are primarily underrated yet they are some of the best foods for weight loss and they also promote optimal health. Although it has a lot of carbs, potassium is a vital element that is present in potatoes. This potassium is important as it controls the blood pressure levels. Many people who were stranded in desolate places such as islands, claimed to live on potatoes and other roots for extended periods of time. What's more, potatoes also ranked highest on the satiety index – which measures how filling different food items are. To ensure optimum weight loss, the trick is to boil the potatoes and cool it for a while so that it forms a large amount of resistant starch – which is a fibre like substance that has all sorts of health benefits. You could also remain guilt free and consume sweet potatoes, turnips and other root vegetables like yam.

- Beans

High in both- protein and fibre, legumes such as kidney beans, lentils, moong, and black beans are healthy and promote weight loss. They also consist of some amount of resistant starch.

- Soups

It is a good idea to consume soups for dinner or for supper because they tend to ensure that you eat fewer calories. You can make a soup out of any vegetable that you like. Because the bulk of the soup is water and some essential ingredients, you really do not have to worry about the chances of calorie gain.

- Cottage Cheese

This is welcoming news for all the cheese lovers. It has been scientifically proven that cottage cheese is high in protein – meaning that it has very little carbohydrate and fat. Besides being healthy, it is also easy to make and can be made at home or brought at the stores. It keeps you feeling satiated and happy despite having eaten a limited quantity.

- Avocados

Avocados are among the most unique and highly nutritious fruits. This fruit contains healthy fats especially the monounsaturated oleic acid which is also found in olive oils. The presence of water in the avocados ensures that they are not as dense as other fruits and they also contain sufficient quantities of fibre and potassium. They complement salads too and they can be eaten as it is as fruit servings. If you aren't minding your waistline, then it is best to have a scoop of avocado fruit with a bit of vanilla ice cream.

- Apple Cider Vinegar

Few ingredients in the kitchen are as useful as the apple cider vinegar. You can use it to dress your salads or as vinaigrettes. Diluting it in water and consuming it early morning is not a bad idea either. It also works by reducing the blood sugar spikes after meals.

- Nuts And Dry Fruits

Nuts are the best snacks for your mid-meal munchies because of the healthy blend of nutrition contained in them. Nuts have the right amount of protein, fibre and healthy fats that are not fattening. It is a good idea to keep a few nuts such as almonds, cashews, peanuts or walnuts in an air-tight container so as to much on them when you are at work.

- Whole Grains

Oats, Quinoa and brown rice have become recent diet fads owing to their non-gluten, fibre-rich appeal. Because these whole grains are rich in protein as well, there are plenty of takers for the same. Brown rice contains significant amount of resistant starch, especially when it is cooked and allowed to cool for a while. Oats are gaining popularity as breakfast items – they may be the next cereals. Oats are rich in beta-glucans which are soluble fibre that have been shown to increase satiety and improve metabolic health. Eating grains may not work in your favour if you are on a low-carb diet but it is a good idea to have the healthier versions than the gluten-rich grains.

- Chilli Pepper

Capsaicin is a compound that is contained in chili peppers that may be an effective antidote to weight gain. Capsaicin works by reducing your appetite while you increasing the fat burning ability although this may be debatable in the instances of people who are tolerant towards spicy food.

Everything is acceptable by the body as long as it is within certain limits. You cannot fool your body and consume the junk without realizing that it is going to take a toll on you. Another important thing to remember is that it is all right to take occasional breaks from your diets and exercise regimen. Even if you end up overeating, do not feel guilty about it. Keep working hard and control your portions and you will manage to work off those accidental extra calories too. Just remember to stay away from crash dieting because it will do no good to you and you may end up binge eating after the period of crash dieting.

How Should Your Sample Diet Look Like?

Here is a sample diet that you can follow if it matches your culinary tastes. It would be a great idea to kickstart your ay with a bowl of yoghurt and fruits. There's nothing better than whole fruits and fresh yoghurt. After around two or three hours, you can have a cup of tea or coffee. This will stimulate you and allow you to concentrate on work, especially if the travel to your workplace is a long and hassling commute. The antioxidants present in the coffee will enable you to get a good amount of nutrition. For lunch, a high-protein meal will be great but you can also have salads and stuff. Getting sufficient amounts of fibre will work in your favor and keep you healthy for a longer time.

It is extremely vital to drink a minimum of 8 glasses of water in a day. You have to increase your water consumption if you tend to sweat a lot of if you are living in a warm place. Pace the water consumption throughout your day and do not wait until you feel thirsty. After lunch, your next snack can be a bowl of fruit. Seasonal fruits that are readily available are best for your body – they are naturally great for metabolism as well. Nature has a way of complementing the season with the choicest of fruits and you must have these fresh fruits rather than the frozen supplements of non-seasonal fruits. A bowl of grapes, some diced mango, apple slices, banana chops, all of these are great food ideas for snack breaks.

Dinner must be lighter than the other meals that you consume throughout the day. It is a great idea to eat sea food such as salmon, lobster or shellfish. If you are craving for some white meat, then chicken is also a perfect substitute. Try to avoid carbs like rice or flat bread during dinner. A warm glass of milk never hurts and gives credence to the old wife's story of getting a good night's rest. Sleep is an underrated element of your day. You have to get enough rest for your body to rejuvenate and your cells to heal. Sleep gives your body time to catch up and your mind usually needs at least six hours of sleep per day. If you find that you are not sleeping enough and it is exceedingly difficult to go to bed, then you should increase your activity levels. You may need to expend more energy in order to get tired.

Non-Exercise Activity Thermogenesis or NEAT as it is called lately is another way to increase the calorie burn count of your metabolism. What you can do is ensure that you keep your body busy with little activities like stretching, climbing instead of using the lift, or walking about as you talk on the phone. Just a few small lifestyle adjustments can help you lose as much as 350 calories per day.

Chapter 7: Exercise Heartily

There are simple tips to boost your metabolism for up to 24 hours post-exercise by adding just one little twist to your exercise routine. Try and add brief periods of intense effort into your regular workouts. If you are adept at walking on an everyday basis, then you could try to or runs, swim, or cycle for a shorter duration.

Truth be told, exercise may, in fact, be more important for women than it is for men. This is because a woman's body undergoes several changes and it is essential that the hormonal imbalance is adjusted by various manners and exercise is primary among them.

Exercising is a routine activity that helps women stay busy and this helps one be independent at least physically because it helps keeps your heart healthy and elevates your heart rate and breathing.

Exercise is the best stress reliever ever and regardless of the root of your frustration, when you exercise, you give vent to a lot of feelings that finally find the right outlet. You could go for a walk at the bay or hit the gym in full stead, all that pent-up energy can be put to use and you will feel better instantly.

It is a good way of showing kids that exercise is essential. It can improve your self-discipline in various ways and teach kids the same.

Women are more prone to diseases like osteoporosis and this can be countered by lifting weights, running, yoga or regular aerobics. It also lowers the occurrence of type 2 diabetes and cancers besides regulating blood pressure level.

Fitness should be a priority for women from their early twenties itself to get them into the right lifestyle attitudes. There are other exercises like pilates, kickboxing or Zumba for the people who love fun workouts. Varying workouts are great for the body as different muscles are put to use at different times and there is no lull.

Exercising releases a lot of feel-good hormones also called endorphins. If nothing, at least this should be your motivation to work out regularly. If you are feeling a bout of depression, then there is no better way to treat it yourself than to keep your body and mind focussed on your health. Increased levels of fitness will actually lift your mood and allow you to sleep better in the night and this is a good start to your body. These endorphins are hormones are released into the bloodstream and their effects are so positive that it will energize you instantly. You do not need to spend hours together sweating it out at the gym, just commit at least half an hour of your day to working out and things will look a lot better for you.

Aerobics are a fun-filled way of working out and it allows you to try different variations too. You could play your favorite music and even groove to myriad funky tunes in order to exercise to your heart's content. Aerobics can help women lose weight faster, especially when done in a group. Peer pressure contributes to this and one can even enjoy the process or bonding that occurs with other people when exercising.

Lift Weights

Sporadic, improper dieting may often cause muscle loss and metabolic slowdown. It is also referred to as the starvation mode. Lifting weights can help you keep your muscle mass intact as it is a form of resistance exercise.

The intensity of these short bursts of exercise effectively resets your metabolism to a slightly higher rate during your workout session. For example, if you're a regular walker and you typically exercise for 20 minutes, then you should try and jog for 60 seconds every 10 minutes. The duration can be increased as and when you progress through the exercise intensity. They say that exercising is like a drug and the only side effects of this drug are good looks. If you think about it, this adage actually makes a lot of sense and it may even inspire you to take up the workouts head on.

Some of the workout regimens you can focus on including the following:

Understanding Push ups

One of the best exercises that you can add to your repertoire of workouts includes push ups. Regardless of what you are training for – whether it is muscle growth, general fitness, weight loss or strength training, your fitness guru is sure to make you do a couple of these exercises. Push ups help you burn calories and boosts endurance levels. This targets your chest, shoulders, and triceps, mainly the upper body strength. Although it varies according to the positioning of the hand and foot of different people, one normally lifts at least 70 percent of their body weight if push ups are done the right way. Hence on some levels, it may actually be better than curls or lateral raises. Push ups are great metabolism boosters too. Since the focus is on the upper body, you must allow your back and leg muscles to be exercised in a different way. It would be a good idea to combine push-ups with other intensity workouts for better results if you are looking exclusively at weight loss as the final result. Combine it with a good amount of cardio, crunches, lunges, and squats for effective weight loss.

Understanding Crunches

Crunches and sit-ups are said to burn calories in the navel area but it also helps in general weight loss. It takes a lot more energy to do crunches so you end up burning more calories too. If you are doing crunches as a part of your fitness plan, you should start with the basics and then include variations as you go along.

For a fitness program to be effective, you have to realize that it's going to take a while for the results to be visible. Unlike the marks you get in exams, you cannot quantify the results of exercising and dieting immediately. You have to cultivate a positive outlook and work on your patience. If you have out in enough effort, then the results will show off your determination and you will be extremely happy with it.

Chapter 9: What Food Items Should You Stay Away From?

Trans fats

Trans fats are everything that is wrong with junk food regardless of which form of junk you are consuming. Fries, pizzas, cookies, cakes, and even your favorite hamburger usually contain some additives and trans fats that make it harmful for consumption on a regular basis. The use of hydrogenated cooking oil causes a lot of cholesterol that indirectly shows its effects on your clothes.

Sugar

On the whole, do not obsess over the quantity of sugar that you may have mistakenly consumed. It is okay to eat low-fat, high-fibre foods that may have a little amount of sugar content. Moderation is the key to healthy eating and you will benefit if you follow this on a daily basis. It's not just sugar that you have to be wary of. Make it a point to stay away from hot chips as well because potato crisps, cheese dips, corn chips etc are things that you may over eat without even realizing it, especially if you are at the movies.

Refined flour

Pizzas are no less dangerous to your weight loss regimen. Most pizza bases constitute refined flour which is bad for people who are trying to diet. Crackers with cheese are other culprits that you must be wary of. Refined flour is generally stripped of the fibrous elements and hence they can spike your blood sugar levels rapidly. This may leave you hungrier than you were.

Artificial Sweeteners

There is a surge in the availability of artificial sweeteners in the market owing to the emphasis of sugar on our health. However, if you thought that artificial sweeteners are the solution to your health issues, you could not be more wrong. The most common sugar substitute is actually aspartame and overconsumption of this can lead to a host of serious issues like insomnia, depression, blindness, and in rare cases, even Alzheimer's. In a move to include all fitness freaks, aspartame is actually extensively present in all sugar-free items such as aerated drinks, pastries, yoghurt, ice-creams, or even cereals. Ensure that kids are never given foodstuffs containing aspartame as it can impair their natural development.

The thing about aspartame is that it leaves an aftertaste in the tongues and this often fools your mind into believing that you're thirsty, making you end up drink more carbonated beverage or salty foods to complement the taste. In the process, you will actually end up consuming more than you intended to.

High Fructose Corn Syrup

High Fructose Corn Syrup is actually a sweetener that makes you crave more sugar. It is used generously in aerated drinks like Coca-cola, Pepsi, and 7UP. What's more, even your favorite brand of flavored yoghurt may have this as a primary ingredient to add that tinge of flavor. It is best to stick to pure, unadulterated water when you're super thirsty. If you want some flavors, then having fresh juice is a better option than relying on the soda fizz.

Monosodium Glutamate

Commonly referred to as MSG or Ajinomoto, this is a common ingredient in almost all Chinese recipes. If you have always wondered why the noodles taste so much better at the restaurant than all your attempts at making the perfect noodles, then it is not your culinary skills that must be questioned. The answer to that lies in the extensive use of MSG at the stores. You will have to be a little smart in identifying whether your food contains MSG as it may be disguised as textured protein, yeast extract, or mono-potassium glutamate.

Now that you are aware of these killer chemicals, avoid these like the plague and you will be better off without its insidious effects.

Chapter 10: Miscellaneous Questions And Answers

Why You Should Chew Slowly?

Although this may sound weird, it is important to chew slowly as it fools the brain into thinking that it has had enough. You may even end up getting tired of all the chewing and actually consume fewer calories on the whole.

Why you must Stay Strong?

Your addiction for certain non-healthy food stuff will always get you if you do not remain firm. You must aim to be strong willed and control your cravings from over-powering you. Keep reminding yourself of all the consequences of the results. If you eat it without meaning to, you will increase your calorie count. Do you really want that to happen? If the answer is a no, then go right ahead and ignore the craving.

Why is brushing important?

This may sound downright stupid but the thing is, if you are the kind of person who gets the strangest cravings around midnight, you may need to eat more during your dinners. In case you still suffer from the irritating habit of hunger pangs when you end up munching on processed and packaged foodstuffs like biscuits, it would help you if you followed this trick.

If you are sure that you do not want to eat anything beyond a specific time, then make sure that you brush your teeth everyday around the said amount of time. The minty aftertaste of the paste will discourage you from thinking about all the food that you can try.

Why should you say No to diets?

Dieting should not be a solution to weight loss, dieting should mean identifying the kind of foodstuffs that you like and that which will ensure that you remain healthy. Cutting some food items on the pretext of them being fattening or filling is not the way it is supposed to work. People who actually leave out a lot of nutritious food suffer because of this. Instead of going on a crash diet, losing kilos, being unable to maintain it and piling on more kilos, it would be more apt to nourish your body with the right kind of food to keep it going. Celebrity influences may tempt you into trying the latest fads like green juices, pumpkin, grape or papaya diets but stay away from these!

Conclusion

To conclude, all the pointers present in this book will be void if you yourself do not intend to lose weight and remain fit. The goal of your exercises and eating habits must actually be about getting fit. Also, remember this, the best motivation to lose weight is when you want to do it for yourself. However, if you keep finding reasons to remain lazy, then you have to agree to the consequences. It might help to have a role model in your mind. A role model, in this case, is someone who inspires you to challenge your limits and bring out the best of your abilities.

You do not always have to look at celebs to be your role models. If you are a huge fan of Jenifer Lopez, Maria Sharapova, Sofia Vergara or Salma Hayek, then you should understand that they look like a million dollars because they sweat it out every single day and control their diets extensively. Your peers or friends may also be your role models as long as they continue to inspire you every day with their motivation and support. It is a good idea to find a support group within your friends who can help keep a check on your eating habits as well as workouts. You could also motivate each other to continue working hard every day with a common goal. Our goal could be as varied as fitting into an old, favorite dress, running a marathon, climbing a hill, or anything that challenges and excites you. Keep going strong until you both see the light of day and celebrate your much-deserved success with your support group.

Thank you so much for downloading this book. I do hope you feel motivated and ready to achieve your fitness goals.

If you enjoyed reading this book, I would really appreciate if you could leave a review.

Thanks!

www.ingramcontent.com/pod-product-compliance
Lightning Source LLC
Chambersburg PA
CBHW061950280526
45787CB00004B/1800